PALEO ~~~~ LIST

Paleo Food Shopping List for the Supermarket

Diet Grocery list of Vegetables, Meats, Fruits and Pantry Foods

by Jane Burton

Published by Kangaroo Flat Books

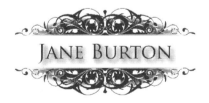

JANE BURTON

- VISIT THE AUTHOR'S PAGE -

http://www.amazon.com/author/janeburton

ISBN-13: 978-1500136277

ISBN-10: 1500136271

❧❦

TABLE OF CONTENTS

PALEO FOOD SHOPPING LIST..................................7

PALEO PANTRY LIST...9

NON STARCHY VEGETABLES..............................11

PALEO VEGETABLE LIST 13

PALEO FRESH FRUIT LIST....................................15

PALEO DRIED FRUITS..17

PALEO MEATS..19

PALEO FRESH MEAT LIST...............................20

PALEO SEAFOOD LIST...21

EGGS ARE PALEO!...22

PALEO NUT & SEED LIST.....................................23

PALEO CONDIMENTS 25

PALEO HERBS 27

NOTES 28

PALEO SPICES 29

PALEO OIL & BUTTER LIST 31

PALEO NON DAIRY LIST 33

AVOID DAIRY FOODS......................................36

AVOID LEGUMES 36

AVOID FOODS WITH SALTS 37

AVOID FATTY MEATS......................................37

AVOID SOFT DRINKS & SUGARY FRUIT JUICES 38

AVOID JUNK FOODS! 38

PALEO DIET & FREE RECIPE BOOKS 38

FREE GIFT 41

COPYRIGHT 43

Download and print off your Free Meal Planner and Shopping List at the web address below.

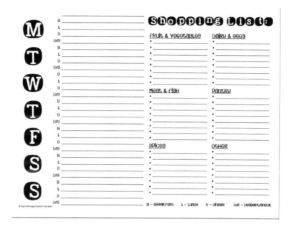

http://paleorecipeblog.com

PALEO FOOD SHOPPING LIST

ഇ) C೪

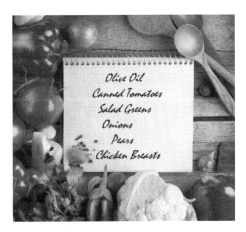

This Paleo shopping list is a guide you can quickly access when out shopping. We have all been caught in the supermarket unsure if something is Paleo or not. Download and print off the meal planner and shopping list if that makes things quicker and easier. Although every food in the supermarket can't be listed, most commonly found Paleo foods are here. So if I've missed a few, my apologies for that. **If you are unsure, ask yourself the question - is it natural?** Check the labels. Ask the butcher where the meat comes from or how it is prepared. If you can't find a particular Paleo food at the supermarket, don't give up, try the health food store! It's better to stick to the Paleo diet and eat "regular" non Paleo until you find something else to take its place. A general rule of thumb I use is to be wary of packaged foods. Happy shopping!

Once you get the idea of the Paleo diet, you won't need this list as much. I didn't want this book to be cluttered and difficult to find things on the list, so for this reason it doesn't have details about the Paleo diet here. For more in depth information check out my "Paleo Diet for Modern People" book on Amazon here at www.amazon.com/author/janeburton

Stock your trolley up on any favorite items you see on special. Plan to have a cook up if something you like is on sale in the fruit, vegetable and meat section. You can always freeze the leftovers. Depending on the layout of your supermarket, let's start with the Pantry items first.

PALEO PANTRY LIST

℘℘℘

General items for the pantry: What's in your pantry? If it isn't looking very Paleo friendly, don't worry, in time you'll get it into shape! Read the Food Nutrition labels to spot non Paleo ingredients.

- Eggs
- Baking Soda
- Almond Flour
- Almond Meal
- Coconut Flour
- Arrowroot Powder (some say it's fine, others say no. Use in moderation for thickening stews etc)
- Canned Tomatoes or fresh organic (in moderation)
- Apple Cider Vinegar (Raw)
- Balsamic Vinegar
- Red Wine Vinegar
- Organic Tomato Ketchup (not recommended, but If you must use it, Heinz do an organic one)
- Dijon Mustard
- Horseradish
- Anchovy Paste
- Coconut Aminos (soy sauce substitute)
- Capers
- Pine Nuts
- Pumpkin Seeds
- Sunflower Seeds
- Sesame Seeds
- Chia Seeds
- Natural Sesame Seed Paste (Tahini)
- Anchovy Paste
- Natural Stock
- Olive Oil (extra virgin best)

- Coconut Oil
- Avocado Oil
- Macadamia Oil
- Walnut Oil
- Sesame Seed Oil
- Coffee Beans (whole or ground – in moderation)
- Tea Leaves (organic, herbal best – standard in moderation)
- Dark 85%+ Cocao Chocolate
- 100% Cocao Powder
- Water (rain or natural)
- Coconut Milk
- Coconut Cream (in moderation)
- Coconut Water
- Capers
- Butter (grass fed, organic)
- Almond Milk (I use SoGood)
- Almond Butter
- Cashew Butter
- Fresh Nuts (Almond, Walnut, Pecans, Macadamia, Cashews, Hazelnuts, raw, unsalted)
- Dried Fruits
- Salt (sea or rock)
- Black Pepper
- Organic natural Honey
- Organic Dates make great sweeteners when cooking
- Prunes make a good snack or as a sweetener when cooking
- Agave Nectar, Stevia, Maple Sugar or Coconut Sugar if you must, but only in moderation
- Herbs & Spices see below

NON STARCHY VEGETABLES

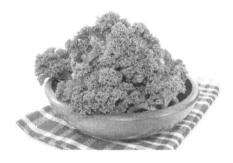

Non starchy veggies like all leafy greens, broccoli, kale, cauliflower, capsicum peppers, cucumbers, carrots, mushrooms, and celery are a good option for weight loss. Non starchy vegetables are full of vitamins, minerals, fiber and phytochemicals, but with few calories. The goal of the Paleo diet is every bite of food you eat provides a generous dose of nutrients or some type of health benefit. **Making homemade juice is another way I get nutrients into the body fast.** My family enjoys the vegetable spiked drinks too! Learn about the overlooked powers of healthy juices in my juicer recipes book.

Paleo Vegetables - Common Starchy Vegetables

If you want to lose weight or remove toxins from your body quickly, be very strict only eating Paleo foods, say for about 30 days. Also reduce starchy veggies and fruits during this time. Then slowly add a few Paleo foods that can be eaten in moderation. Vegetables high in starch can raise blood sugar levels compared to non starchy types, so people with diabetes can look at limiting their intake too. **Common higher starch vegetables include potatoes, peas, corn and yams. Sweet potato and yams are Paleo but eat in moderation.**

PALEO VEGETABLE LIST

ഔഌ

On the Paleo diet for weight loss these non starchy vegetables are the most recommended. Eat them raw, steamed, cooked with other foods, for baking or in Paleo smoothies. **Organic is best.** When shopping look for fresh in season, organic varieties if available. **Can't go wrong with most veggies except white potatoes, peas, corn and beans...load the trolley up!** They are healthy and full of vitamins and fibre. Wash and peel if appropriate. Source locally if possible or grow your own. Potatoes contain anti-nutrients like saponins that can be harmful, while sweet potatoes don't contain these substances. Sweet potato is quite high in carbs though, so limit their use in recipes.

- Artichoke
- Asparagus
- Avocado (technically a fruit)
- Broccoli
- Brussels Sprouts
- Garlic
- Mushroom
- Broccoli
- Carrots
- Cauliflower
- Bell pepper (red, yellow, green)
- Beets (in moderation for weight loss)
- Cabbage(red & white, Chinese, collard greens)
- Celery
- Cauliflower
- Carrots (raw has lower GI)
- Cucumber
- Chard
- Cucumber
- Dandelion Greens

- Eggplant
- Fennel root
- Kale
- Lettuce
- Onion
- Pumpkin
- Parsnip
- Parsley
- Radish
- Salad greens (all)
- Seaweed
- Spinach
- Spring onions
- Sweet potato (in moderation for weight loss)
- Squash (in moderation for weight loss)
- Tomato (technically a fruit - avoid if you have autoimmune problems - only in moderation - nightshade)
- Turnip
- Zucchini

PALEO FRESH FRUIT LIST

 හොශ

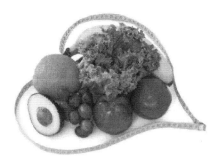

Let's move on to the fruit section of the supermarket next! All fruit is good on a Paleo diet but they do have high sugar levels so eat in moderation. If you want to lose weight limit to about 2 serves a day. high sugar fruits (grapes, bananas, mangoes, sweet cherries, apples, pineapples, pears and kiwi fruit - while Berries, watermelon, cantaloupe, mango, peaches, grapefruit, oranges, plums, apples and bananas are good. Fruit is natural, healthy and a good source of vitamins and fibre. Try to buy organic fruit in season. Wash and if in doubt peel to remove any possible chemical residue. Source locally if possible.

- Apple
- Apricot
- Avocado (a favorite - great for cooking and salads)
- Banana
- Blackberries
- Blueberries
- Boysenberries

- Cranberries
- Cherimoya
- Cantaloupe
- Carambola (star fruit)
- Cherries
- Casaba Melon
- Figs
- Gooseberries
- Grapefruit
- Grapes
- Guava
- Honeydew melon
- Kiwi
- Lemons
- Limes
- Lychee
- Mango
- Nectarine
- Orange
- Passion Fruit
- Papaya
- Peaches
- Pears
- Persimmon
- Pomegranate
- Pineapple
- Raspberries
- Rhubarb
- Star Fruit
- Strawberries
- Tangerine
- Tomato (avoid if you have autoimmune problems)
- Watermelon

Paleo Dried Fruits

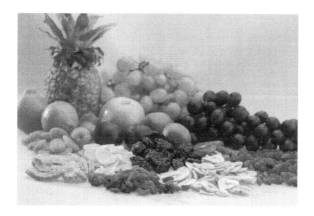

Eat dried fruits in moderation due to their high carb/sugar content. A handful of mixed fruit and nuts a day is good. Consider drying fruit yourself using no preservatives and store in jars. This is wonderful on the years my fruit trees bear plenty of fruit. Bananas can be hard to digest, so eat in moderation. Remember that whole dried fruits can have less sugar than small pieces. Cranberries are a good example of this.

- Apple
- Apricot
- Bananas
- Blackberries
- Blueberries
- Cantaloupe
- Cranberries
- Pears

- Figs
- Goji Berries
- Grapes (sultanas white, currants dark)
- Lychee
- Lemon
- Lime
- Mango
- Nectarine
- Papaya
- Peaches
- Plums (dates)
- Raspberries
- Strawberries
- Watermelon
- Pineapple Guava
- Tangerine
- Oranges

PALEO MEATS

৯০৫৪

Now let's move on to the meat department. Check out specials, the quality of the meat and how fresh it looks/use by date. A nice pinkish color means it's fresh. The following meats are allowed on the Paleo diet. **You'll need to avoid all processed meats** as they are usually high in nitrates and other chemicals used for preserving. If you can find naturally smoked products such as Chorizos or fish, they are okay. It gets back to the "natural" issue. When buying fish, check the eye is "clear" not "cloudy" suggesting it's fresh.

For weight watchers buy lean meat or trim off all fat. Use little or no oil if frying, try grilling to cook instead. Use olive oil or other recommended oils below. Grass fed meats are Paleo. Pasture fed stock under natural conditions is best. Ask the butcher where the meat came from.

Deli Meats:

Cold sliced quality NATURAL meats from the cold deli section of the supermarket are okay in moderation, only if they are free from preservatives and additives. Only buy NON processed and try to keep them lean if wanting to lose weight. Look for sliced pork, beef, chicken and turkey. Ask the deli assistant what ingredients are in them. Great for Paleo lunches with salad or veg. Naturally processed Chorizos are about the only sausage I know of, but ask your local butcher.

Fresh Meats:

Try to source local, grass fed quality meats if they are available. If not at least look for good quality lean cuts. A little quality goes a long way! Trim excess fat if you are watching your weight. Chuck or stewing steak is the tastiest in slow cooking.

PALEO FRESH MEAT LIST

- Bacon (lean "eye" short cut for weight watchers)
- Beef (grass fed stewing, ground, T-bone, sirloin etc, remove excess fats if required.)
- Chicken Breast (remove excess fats and skin)
- Chicken Leg
- Chicken Thigh
- Chicken Wings
- Emu
- Goat
- Goose
- Kangaroo
- Lamb Chops
- Lamb rack
- Lean Veal
- Ostrich
- Pheasant
- Pork (Fillets, Chops, Tenderloin Steaks etc; trim excess fat)
- Quail
- Rabbit
- Snake
- Steak
- Turkey
- Turtle
- Veal
- Venison
- Wild Boar

PALEO SEAFOOD LIST

ഇ⊃ᲝᲚ

Fish is a good source of Omega 3 oils and very healthy for our bodies. If frying, use a little olive oil or other Paleo friendly oil. It is thought that larger fish may have higher mercury levels which aren't good for our health. Sardines in spring water or olive oil are a great addition for lunches with onion, baby spinach and avocado. This is a basic list, but virtually anything wild caught goes!

- Bass
- Barramundi
- Cod
- Clams
- Crab
- Crawfish
- Crayfish
- Eel
- Flathead
- Halibut
- Lobster
- Mackerel
- Oysters
- Perch
- Prawns (shrimp)
- Whiting
- Salmon
- Sardines
- Shark
- Shrimp
- Snapper
- Scallops
- Tuna

EGGS ARE PALEO!

Nature's little power packs! Poached, hard boiled, omelettes, scrambled, raw in smoothies....the list goes on. Eggs are great for lunches too. Free range is best. If possible, try to buy your eggs where the chickens roam free and have a natural diet. If you have chickens in your own back yard, that is even better. You get eggs and compost for the garden as well as getting rid of your foods scraps!

Eggs: (chicken, duck, quail & goose)

Paleo Nut & Seed List

൧

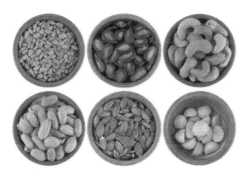

Nuts and Seeds are a great source of "the good oils" Raw, unsalted are best. Again, check the labels.

- Almonds
- Cashews
- Hazelnuts
- Macadamia
- Pecans
- Pistachio (unsalted, in moderation)
- Walnuts
- Sunflower Seeds
- Sesame Seeds
- Pumpkin Seeds (Pepitas)

PALEO CONDIMENTS

৯৩৫৪

Always check labels on the packaging. Think natural - no preservatives, additives, artificial flavors etc. Beware "blends" with additives and high salt or fat content. Mixed natural herbs are okay, fresh is better again. Grow some in your own garden. If you don't have space, use pots. That's what I do.

Olive oil, avocado and Dijon is very versatile and can be used for many things like over a salad, cooking etc. Quality red wine vinegar, apple cider vinegar, balsamic vinegar and even natural ketchup may be found depending on your local store. Have a look to see what's available on the shelves and read the ingredients label. The supermarket or health food store may have items for special diets. One of the best basic salad dressings I use is olive oil with a squeeze of fresh lemon juice. Mashed Avocado is wonderful too!

- Apple Cider Vinegar
- Balsamic Vinegar
- Red Wine Vinegar
- Dijon Mustard
- Coconut Aminos (soy sauce substitute)
- Homemade dressing (fresh lemon & olive oil**)**

PALEO HERBS

ഇറ്റ

Fresh herbs are tasty nutrient packed little wonders. **Think organic...anything goes.** If you are lucky enough to grow your own herbs, that is fabulous!

My favorite herbs in pots are parsley, chives, coriander, rosemary and basil. I have even managed to find a basil-mint cross...great in curries! Dried herbs are good too and add interest to foods.

- Basil
- Bay leaf
- Chives
- Cardamom
- Cilantro (Coriander)
- Celery Seed
- Dill
- Fennel
- Mint
- Oregano
- Rosemary
- Parsley
- Paprika
- Thyme
- Marjoram

Notes

PALEO SPICES

Where would the world be without spices! Anything goes.

- Allspice
- Black Pepper
- Curry
- Chili Powder (red, yellow & green)
- Cayenne Pepper
- Cardamom
- Celery Seed
- Cinnamon
- Cumin
- Fenugreek
- Garlic (flakes, natural powder)
- Garam Masala
- Ginger
- Nutmeg
- Paprika
- Natural Salt (in moderation)
- Star Anise
- Turmeric

Paleo Oil & Butter List

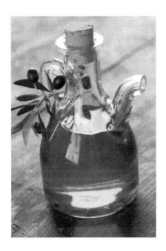

Did you know oils like flaxseed oil are good for your hair (makes it healthy and shiny) and nails too?

Don't forget butters and oil are high in fat and calorie content, so go easy if you are trying to lose weight.

Oils:

- Olive Oil
- Avocado Oil
- Almond Oil
- Flaxseed Oil
- Walnut Oil
- Coconut Oil
- Macadamia Oil
- Sesame Seed Oil

Butters:

- Grass Fed Butters Only

- Almond Butter
- Fat - Lard
- Ghee
- Coconut Butter
- Cashew Butter

Paleo Non Dairy List

৩০৫

While some people are concerned about not getting enough calcium while eating Paleo foods, following a healthy diet with a variety of nutritious foods will give you as much calcium as you need. As an example, sardines and spinach are very high in calcium...who would have thought! Sardines and salad makes for a wonderful lunch. Calcium depletion and lack of absorption can occur through bad diet and an unhealthy lifestyle which can be even more damaging.

*Look for unsweetened, unflavored milks.

- Coconut Milk*
- Coconut Cream
- Almond Milk*
- Almond Butter
- Cashew Butter
- Grass Fed Butter

AVOID GRAINS

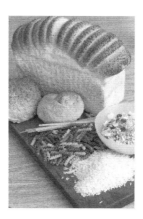

Grains are in most of our breakfast cereals and breads today. They are usually highly processed and have added sugars and additives in them. Avoid all products associated with these base grains. Gluten free is good, but avoiding all grain is better if you are strict Paleo. At least reduce it dramatically...see the effect on your tummy and digestion, it will love you for it! (Flaxseeds are good if you are into Paleo breads) Eating less carbs will also help you reduce weight.

- Barley
- Corn
- Couscous
- Millet
- Oats
- Rice
- Rye
- Sorghum
- Wheat
- Amaranth
- Buckwheat
- Quinoa

Avoid Dairy Foods

All dairy products including processed products are to be avoided.
Sadly most supermarket dairy products are heavily processed and
altered today. Use almond milk or coconut milk/cream instead of
cow's milk as a staple. A balanced diet and healthy lifestyle will
maintain your calcium levels.

Avoid Legumes

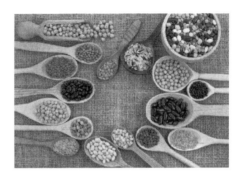

**Basically put, legumes contain Lectins, which may irritate and be
a problem for the stomach. This includes peanuts.**

- All beans
- Black - eyed peas
- Chickpeas
- Lentils
- Peas
- Miso
- Peanut butter
- Peanuts
- Snow peas
- Sugar snap peas
- Soybeans and all soybean products, including tofu
- Starchy Vegetables
- Starchy tubers
- Cassava
- Manioc
- Potatoes (except sweet potato)
- Tapioca pudding

AVOID FOODS WITH SALTS

Almost all commercial salad dressings and condiments are unhealthy. Read the labels! If you can source natural, low salt unprocessed products then go for it! You can trying making your own! Bacon is allowed on the Paleo diet but common sense should prevail as it can be very salty and high in fats. Only eat in moderation if weight loss is the aim or cut off excess fat.

- Cheese
- Processed meats
- Frankfurters
- Ham
- Hot dogs
- Ketchup
- Olives
- Pickled foods
- Pork rinds
- Processed canned meats and fish (unless they are unsalted or unless you soak and drain them. Sardines in springwater are good. If in olive oil eat in moderation)
- Salted nuts
- Salami
- Spices blends with salts and additives
- Sausages (naturally made Chorizo may be okay in moderation. Ask your local butcher)
- Dried fish or meat like beef jerky if high in salt. Homemade may be an alternative.

AVOID FATTY MEATS

Avoid Processed Foods & Meats - replace with lean fresh meat. Budget wise, look for specials. Remember a little top quality goes a long way!
Avoid Fatty cuts of beef, pork lamb and any other fat meats. Watch how you cook them too! No point buying a nice lean piece of beef, just to take it home and cook it in loads of vegetable oil! Try to source quality, local grass fed meats or wild caught fish.

AVOID SOFT DRINKS & SUGARY FRUIT JUICES

All sugary canned, bottled and soft drinks (due to additives - they are like tasty poison!) Highly processed juices should be avoided too. **The ingredients list tells all** - generally I find the word "drink" on packaging relates to little fruit, but a whole lot of other stuff - beware as these can have little fibre and high GI! Read the label, you can find some raw, natural, sugar free brands. Another cheap, healthy option is to make your own healthy smoothies or juices. Natural is always the best.

AVOID JUNK FOODS!

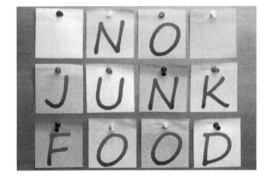

- Sweets
- Candy

All processed Cakes, Biscuits, Bread & Grain Based Products. My Paleo recipe books with almond flour and coconut flour can be found at *www.amazon.com/author/janeburton*

- All Sugars and Sugar Based Products
- Potato Chips

Eat foods where sugar occurs naturally; your body will LOVE you for it!

Paleo Diet & Free Recipe Books

Get a Free copy of my Paleo Desserts book here
http://paleodessertsandtreats.com

If you would like full color books, my Paleo Kindle books are often free or on sale, so go to *www.amazon.com/author/janeburton* to view them. Here are the book titles –

- *Paleo Diet for Weight Loss*
- *Almond Flour Cookbook*
- *Paleo Smoothies*
- *Paleo Recipes for Busy People*
- *Coconut Milk Recipes*
- *Paleo Crockpot Cookbook*
- *Kale Cookbook*
- *Make Ahead Paleo*
- *Lunch Box Recipes*
- *Paleo Appetizers*
- *7 Day Paleo Meal Plan*

Read more about nutrients in foods at the US Nutrients Database here at *http://ndb.nal.usda.gov.* Happy shopping and I hope this staple Paleo list of foods helps you get through the checkout more quickly and home to prepare your healthy Paleo meals!

If this book has helped you with your grocery shopping please leave a review, thanks!

http://www.amazon.com/review/create-review

FREE GIFT

As a valued customer I want to send you a free gift :) You can download the book at the address below. I hope you enjoy it! Remember...sweets in moderation.

Please share with your friends if you think they may like it too.

http://paleodessertsandtreats.com

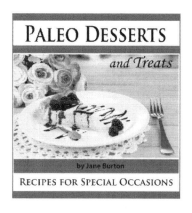

Thanks, I hope you enjoyed this book and our paths cross again in another of my books!

ℰℭ

The End

SHOPPING LIST NOTES

COPYRIGHT

Printed in Great Britain
by Amazon